How To Grow A Beard FAST!

All You Need To Know About Growing And Grooming Sexy Facial Hair

Table of Contents

INTRODUCTION

As if by conspiracy, boys are encouraged to shave off their beards as soon as they start growing them. Beards have become a sort of a taboo (for lack of a better term). Shave for your first date, shave for your graduation speech, shave for your job interview, and so on.

But the more people are trying to promote the clean shave culture, the timeless beard is also seeing a devoted increase in its fan club.

There is no denying the fact that a well-sported beard is a really special thing. When maintained properly, a beard makes a man stand apart just as effectively as a tailored suit. The best part is that a growing a beard doesn't cost a thing. It's all natural.

In the following chapters, we will reinforce your desire to sport a beard and teach you how to grow it fast!

Why Grow a Beard?

Why not?

Keeping a beard is not an easy thing. It requires daily commitment, and it changes the way you look. Hence, you need to be fully motivated before you start growing that stubble.

Besides the fact that Chuck Norris (and Jesus Christ) sports a beard, here are some major benefits of foregoing the dreaded act of shaving your face clean:

Women Love Beards

Every man has his preferences, but if you want women to respond to you, growing a beard isn't a bad idea. It's more than visual attractiveness. Women love to *touch* men's beard. Depending on the level of interaction, they will go right ahead and run their fingers through your beard.

And if you play your cards right, you can easily turn a *'OMG, how long have your been growing that?'* into a excuse for physical contact by taking her hand and leading it to the beard!

And there is scientific proof to back this up. According to a research published in Evolution & Human Behavior (Dixon and Brooks 2013), *'Facial hair strongly influences people's judgments of men's socio-sexual attributes'* and that in the study 'women judged faces with heavy stubble as most attractive and heavy beards, light stubble and clean-shaven faces as similar less attractive'.

Beard Changes Self-Perception

The beard is associated with a rough 'n' tough lifestyle. You start to develop a new appreciation for your own manliness, which helps a lot in displaying self-confidence. And this positive change in your perception about yourself will transfer to others as well. As you walk strong and tall, others will look upon you as the natural leader in virtually any situation.

The beard gives off a 'been there, done that' impression that leads people to believe that a bearded man always seems to know where he is going.

Its More than Just Manliness

While a beard helps you exude the rugged manly look, it is not the only image associated with the stub. We know that many famous scientists, artists, and especially writers were bearded gentlemen. The list includes people like Leo Tolstoy, Walt Whitman, Fyodor Dostoyevsky, Allen Ginsberg, Ernest Hemingway, and Henry David Thoreau.

As Hemingway wrote in *A Farewell to Arms* 'If any man wants to raise a beard, let him.'

How can we disagree with a Nobel Laureate?

It's the Hottest New Look

Let's face it. A beard looks good on almost all celebrities. Examples include George Clooney, Ben Affleck, Michael Fassbender, Justin Timberlake, Tom Hardy, Chris Hemsworth, and once again, Chuck Norris. The bottom line is that when you decide to grow a beard, you are in good company.

A Lesson from History

Before we move on towards the practical aspects of growing a beard, I want to draw attention towards a fascinating incident on the subject of growing beards that involves the greatest American president (and 3-time Oscar winner), Abraham Lincoln.

Lincoln's legacy is unparalleled in history, and here is the proof.

Back in 1982, more than 4 dozen scholars were asked by a leading newspaper to rate all American presidents, going backwards from Carter, in the following categories:

- Leadership Qualities
- Integrity
- Crisis management
- Political skills
- Appointments

The general consensus was that Abe Lincoln was the nation's greatest President that fulfilled the criteria perfectly. The interesting thing is that during his own time, Lincoln had to fight long and hard to be voted into office. But after his death, he was heralded as the man's man, a savior, a liberator of slaves, and the torchbearer of freedom.

He strived to vindicate democracy and preserve the Union, even if it came at the cost of his own political career. His ultimate victory was the abolishment of slavery.

To achieve this, Lincoln pushed aside various laws. He made war without a declaration of war, and without summoning Congress into special session. He countered Supreme Court opposition by affirming the President's authority as the final interpreter of the Constitution. In short, the guy knew what he was talking about.

But did you know that before stepping into the office, Lincoln was a clean-shaved man? Delegates from his own party often urged him to grow a beard and wear high collars, but he always resisted. But a letter from a certain Grace Bedell changed not only Lincoln's perception, but also history in the process. The letter reads as follows:

Dear Sir

*……………..I am a little girl only eleven years old, but want you should be President of the United States very much so I hope you wont think me very bold to write to such a great man as you are. Have you any little girls about as large as I am if so give them my love and tell her to write to me if you cannot answer this letter. I have got 4 brother's and part of them will vote for you any way and **if you let your whiskers grow I will try and get the rest of them to vote for you you would look a great deal better for your face is so thin. All the ladies like whiskers and they would tease their husband's to vote for you and then you would be President.** My father is a going to vote for you and if I was a man I would vote for you to but I will try and get every one to vote for you that I can I think that rail fence around your picture makes it look very pretty I have got a little baby sister she is nine weeks old and is just as cunning as can be. When you direct your letter direct to Grace Bedell Westfield Chatauque County New York.*

The rest, as they say, is history. When Abraham Lincoln left Springfield in 1861 for the White House, he was fully bearded.

STARTING TO GROW YOUR BEARD

As mentioned before, growing a beard requires commitment as you are essentially making a lifestyle change. It also takes a significant amount of courage, as you know that people may not accept your new look easily.

So, how do you take the first step towards growing facial hair?

Stop Shaving

This is the easiest and most obvious way of growing your beard fast. Just stop shaving and continue this 'no shave' habit for at least a month after you start experiencing beard growth.

A common mistake that most men make is that they start shaping and sculpting their beard during the initial stages of growth. Even if you are aiming to get a special style, you shouldn't touch your beard at all at least for 4 weeks. Just let it grow.

Otherwise, you might cut off too much. Even if all you want is a goatee, let your beard grow uninterrupted, for you can always trim it down later.

After about a month, you can start shaping your beard. This mostly means defining the neck and the cheek line. Our advice is that you leave the beard on the cheeks as it is. Some men shave it off, thereby ruining what could have been an excellent beard. Of course, this depends on how much it grows on your cheeks. For instance, if you feel growth below your eyes, you should consider shaving or sculpting the beard on your cheeks.

The 'neckline', as the name suggests, is at the bottom of your beard around your neck. While you can shape this on your own, it is better to let a barber or a stylist handle it. Check if your current barber or stylist has experience in this style.

Also remember that when you let your beard grow feely, it will not be even and may be a bit unsightly. Hence, it is advised that you grow your beard when there are no formal engagements in the near future.

Plan a Vacation

Yes, you heard that right. Getting a few days away from home, whether for business or for leisure, is one of the best excuses to start growing a beard. If genetics work in your favor, you will start developing stubble after not shaving for 2 to 3 days, but no one will immediately pounce on you because you are travelling.

This is one of the best ways to gain the acceptance of your beard, slowly and gradually. Of course, you shouldn't care about what people think about you in the first place. And as mentioned before, many people (especially women) will actually appreciate your new look.

Moreover, some people don't like beards because they think it makes you resemble terrorists and the homeless! While this is absurd to begin with, there are many ways to trim and maintain a beard that doesn't appear 'uncivil' at all.

You Have to Survive Itching

It is not easy to get used to the hair on your face if you never sported a beard previously. One of the most obvious problems is itching. One of the best ways to control it is by washing the beard area with a gentle shampoo. In addition, you can consider applying baby oil or lotions on the itchy skin. But don't let itching stand in the way of your beard growth.

Do You Need to Shave Every Day?

You must have heard that to grow your beard faster and thicker, you need to shave regularly. Sometimes, even beard enthusiasts repeat this idea. However, for all its worth, this is just a myth like all others. First of all, there is no scientific basis to support this assertion, and if anything, shaving on a frequent basis will reduce the amount of hair that grows on your face and not the other way around.

Hence, the fastest way to grow your beard is to keep it growing without disruption. While certain truth to the fact that hair growth increases faster immediately after you shave, but it's actually decreases soon after.

Caring for your Face

You should take care of your skin and keep it clean in order to stimulate hair growth. You should make it a habit to exfoliate your skin once a week using exfoliate or scrub that is made for men.

A good option in this regard is the exfoliating mask, which you can apply to your face, leave for 10-30 minutes, and then rinse it off. This is necessary to remove dead skin cells that hinder beard growth.

You see, when hair follicles are blocked with dirt or grime, the hair cannot grow. Along with scrubbing the dirt, sweat, and oil off at least twice a day, you should also consider massaging your beard, for the hair follicles are stimulated the same way as the follicles on your scalp. You should consider massaging your face 10-15 minutes at least twice a day.

Also keep your skin clean by washing it with warm water and a mild cleanser twice a day, in the morning and evening. This stimulates the growth of small hair.

Yet another method of caring for your skin is to moisturize it, as this creates a better environment for your beard to grow quickly. But do note that some moisturizing products are better than others when it comes to growing a beard fast. Ideally, you should go for a cream or moisturizer with eucalyptus. Eucalyptus has various benefits. It helps with respiration, killing bacteria, countering effects of aging, and curbing inflammation. Not to mention, it also has a great scent.

You can also use eucalyptus oil, which can be used as:

- Expectorant
- Insecticidal
- Antispasmodic
- Anti-viral
- Anti-infection
- Analgesic
- Anticatarrhal

You can use eucalyptus oil to stimulate the hair follicles. But only use it in small amounts as too much oil can make your facial hair greasy. It is suggested that you use eucalyptus oil an hour or so before bathing, and then use a good shampoo to remove the residue, followed by a good conditioner.

Note: While eucalyptus stimulates hair growth, but you should never apply eucalyptus oil directly to the skin. Instead, dilute it with water or use facial skin care products containing eucalyptus.

Dilute eucalyptus oil by combining four parts water with one part eucalyptus.

You can then apply this solution to your face with a cotton ball and let sit. But if you experience irritation, wash the treatment off immediately and avoid it in the future.

Oil not helps on beard growth, bit ingredients like eucalyptus actually make the beard smell good. Not to mention, it also makes your facial hair healthy and shiny. Natural oils also mimic a man's natural follicle oils so that the skin absorbs them easily. This promotes strong strands.

Ingrown Hair

Finally, you need to check whether there are any ingrown hairs on your face or not, as these hinder the even beard growth on your face. These are hairs that are curled around and they are grown back into your skin instead of rising from it.

This can be due to a hair follicle being clogged by dead skin. As a result, the hair inside it is forced to grow sideways under the skin as compared growing outward in an upward fashion.

Do remember that the growth of ingrown hairs is not a serious issue. It is just that these make growing a beard a bit more difficult.

Ingrown hairs also irritate the skin by producing a raised, red bump that may look like little pimples, and you may even experience painful sores.

These hairs are also itchy and cause discomfort. Pus may also form inside the bumps, causing further discomfort. You may notice these bumps on your cheeks, chin, or neck after you have shaved. This is especially true if you have coarse and curly hair. The latter is more likely to curl around and re-enter the skin, especially following a shave or trimming.

The good thing is that for the most part, ingrown hair goes away on its own. But if it doesn't, ingrown hair can cause infection or create marks on your skin.

Growing a beard is actually a way to avoid ingrown hair. As the beard grows longer, there will be lesser chances of the hair curling around and entering the skin.

Not to mention, most of the tips described above, such as scrubbing your face everyday actually help avoid the growth of ingrown hair. Ideally, you should you should rub your face in a circular motion to weed out ingrown hairs.

There is also a certain way of shaving when you notice ingrown hairs on your face.

To start off, you should wet your skin with warm water and apply a lubricating gel before shaving. Next, shave using a sharp, single-bladed razor and shave in the direction where the hair is growing.

Try to use as few strokes as possible to reduce the chances of hair slipping back into the skin, rinsing the blade after every stroke. Also remember that you don't have to clean shave. Leave a bit of stubble if possible. Likewise, if you are using an electric shaver, don't keep it too close to the skin and hold it just above the surface of your skin. Once you are done, apply a cool washcloth to your skin to reduce irritation.

There are other methods to avoid ingrown hairs, such as the use of depilatory creams that burn off the hair. In addition, hair follicle can also be removed permanently using electrolysis.

Finally, if ingrown hair on your face has become infected, you will require professional help. Your doctor will remove the infected hair by making small cuts in the skin using scalpel or a sterile needle. The doctor may also prescribe medications like antibiotics, retinoids, and steroids.

Get a Beard Comb

It is natural to lose hair. We lose as much as 100 hairs each day. Hence, we have to take care in the early days of the beard growth to avoid additional hair fall. One of the most effective ways to do this is to avoid brushing your beard. A beard comb helps in this regard. As compared to regular comb, it will pull the beard with lesser force, thereby avoiding additional hair loss. Also make it a point to let beard hair fall on its own instead of tugging it out.

Avoid Damaging your Facial Hair

There are some things you have to avoid in order to ensure that your beard grows healthy rapidly. These include not using heat to the style the beard. Also avoid using chemicals on your facial hair.

Any damage to beard is dangerous, because it spreads down to the root. And once the root is damaged, further beard growth is jeopardized.

Additional Tip: While it is great to let your beard grow freely without any interruption, there is no harm in lightly trimming your beard's split ends every 2 months or so. This not only ensures that the ends do not split any further, but that you will also maintain healthy hair for a long, long time.

Using Topical Remedies

- **Minoxidil**

While used mostly for growing hair on your head, there is some evidence to suggest that minoxidil can stimulate facial growth as well. Here is how you can use a bottle of minoxidil.

Squeeze out some foam on your fingers, and gently massage it on your face, especially the areas where you want the beard to grow the most. Do not use more than 1 mL (which would be about ½ capful). Also read the instructions on the bottle to avoid overdose. Not to mention, it is also a good idea to consult your doctor before using minoxidil.

- **Lime and Cinnamon Paste**

Ground Cinnamon and lime are 2 ingredients that can also help you grow beard faster. They can be combined into a thin paste that you can apply to your face.

To make and use the paste:

- Take 2 tbsp of lime and mix it with 1 tbsp.
- Apply this to your face. Keep paste on your face for 25 to 30 minutes
- Rinse it off
- Do this twice a day

However, if you feel any irritation, rinse the paste off immediately.

Another mixture that you can use involves Amla oil and mustard leaves. Amla oil (like jojoba and grape seed oil) is one of the best natural oils to coat the follicles on your beard.

Preparing the paste is easy. Simply mix 3 tablespoons of mustard leaves with ¼ cup Amla oil until paste forms. Apply to your face and let it sit for about 20 minutes.

Rinse the paste off your face. Any unused paste can be kept in the fridge for up to 3 days.

Shampoo for Beard Growth

You are growing facial hair alright, but it is not as thick as you would like it to be. Make sure you following all the techniques mentioned above. However, if the thickness isn't coming rapidly, you can consider using beard growth shampoo.

We refrain from suggesting a brand name. However, there are ingredients that you can look out for. Thee firstly include ketoconazole. This aids beard growth by eliminating fungus that causes beard flaking, eczema, and rashes.

Ketoconazole also ensures that your beard remains free of excess sebum, which is natural oil emanated from hair. Excess sebum can harden into crystal, and if this happens inside or on top of the opening of the follicle, it will not only block the growth of beard hair, but also lead to acne, blackheads, whiteheads, and ingrown hairs.

By dissolving crystallized sebum (and also removing detritus from the hair follicles), ketoconazole leads to an uninterrupted beard growth.

Another ingredient that you should look for in a beard growth shampoo is niacin. This is yet another stimulant that helps proper blood flow to the beard. Niacin is a stimulant that dilates capillaries under the skin, allowing more blood to flow to the follicles. This boost of blood brings much needed nutrients to your beard hair, allowing them to grow thicker, longer, and faster.

Oral Medication

Oral drugs like finasteride can help with beard growth. Finasteride boosts testosterone by up to 20%, which greatly helps with beard growth. However, do remember that this medication is only available via prescription, so only consume it as per the instructions to avoid overdose.

OTHER THINGS THAT HELP BEARD GROWTH

In this section, we will list down things that may not be directly related to your facial hair and skin, but they do help beard growth significantly.

Sleep

Just like muscles, getting plenty of sleep helps your hair grow as well. Even if you have gone past the age of gaining height, the body still uses that capability to grow your hair and repair injuries. Hence, getting adequate rest is one of the first steps in growing your facial hair fast.

In you are in the 15-20 age bracket, then you should try to get 8 hours of sleep every night. Adults can get manage with 6 hours of sleep.

There are plenty of things you can do to get a good night's sleep. Start by ensuring that you have a comfortable mattress to lie on.

Also remove distractions. For instance, people who keep pets at home often allow them to come into the bedroom and even on the bed itself. Avoid this for a while so that you can get uninterrupted sleep. Other people have TV and other electronic devices close by. While these may help you relax, they can interfere with your sleep.

In the first few weeks of your beard growth, you should consider making a sleep schedule i.e. going to bed and getting up at the same time every day, regardless of whether it is a workday or holiday. This consistency improves the body's sleep cycle and boosts the quality of your sleep. You should also consider creating a bedtime ritual, which is a set of activities that signals your body that it's time to sleep. Try things like taking a warm bath, reading, or listening to soothing music.

Of course, this doesn't mean that you start becoming anxious if you don't fall asleep in within 15 minutes. Get and try to do something relaxing until you feel sleepy again.

Exercise

There is a direct link between a healthy body and rapid beard growth. Hence, along with improving your sleep, you should start getting physical exercise as well. If you already hit the gym, nothing can be better.

But if you are not used to working out, getting started isn't such a big deal. You should ideally start cardio exercises like brisk walking or jogging. These don't require any equipment (only good shoes), and they do wonders for your blood flow. Proper blood flow is necessary as it allows any nutrients that you take reach your beard area.

You should start exercising for 25-30 minutes, and only increase the time gradually. Also note that while it is best to work out daily, you can still manage with exercising 4 days a week.

Along with a proper workout, also try to get more active in your life. For instance, prefer the stairs over the elevator when possible, and take your dog out for a walk every day.

Stress-Relief

You may not be able to make the connection, but stress does hinder your efforts of growing a beard fast. And this happens in more than one way.

While several things can account for facial hair loss, alopecia areata, or simply alopecia is a common cause. This medical condition (categorized as an autoimmune disorder) messes with hair growth on the entire body as it is linked with hormonal imbalance.

Of course, you cannot diagnose alopecia yourself. Several tests will be taken, and you will undergo physical examination while your medical history is reviewed. Depending on how serious the hair loss is, hair samples and a skin culture will be taken for a laboratory analysis. In most cases, a skin biopsy is also performed.

There is no definite answer as to what exactly causes the onset of alopecia. In the early stages, beard loss may not be easily identifiable, but as it progresses, you will start to notice serious hair loss, usually in patches. How large the patch is depends on the extent of the hair loss. Also note that if you have strong fingernails, they may start to feel fragile before you start to lose facial hair.

How is all this related to stress? The thing is that while hair loss in alopecia can be diminished with corticosteroid medication (to inhibit immune system activity), and topical medication can be applied to hair growth, this alone may not be enough to treat this condition. You also have to keep your stress levels in check.

On average, we lose about 100 hairs per day, but when we are stressed out, we can lose significantly more. Any stress trigger, such as problems at work or family issues, can escalate beard hair loss.

When stress levels increase, the body's defense mechanism is used to deal with the perceived threat, which means other vital functions (like beard growth) suffer.

Stress also works in a cycle. It increases hair loss, which in turn can make you anxious about your appearance. Just like any medical condition, stress can only be diagnosed by a certified expert and has proper treatments.

But for the most part, you can manage your stress levels on your own. The good news is that by adopting healthy habits like sleeping 6-8 hours every night and working out, you are already minimizing the negative effects of stress on your life.

Eat a Healthy Diet

While there is no specific diet for beard growth, incorporating healthy foods in your diet does boost the speed of your beard growth. To start off, you need to increase the amount of protein in your diet, which means you need to have more meat, fish, eggs, nuts, and beans etc.

How does protein boost hair growth? Well, our hair comprises of keratin. Keratin uses amino acids as its food sources and these in turn are provided by protein. It takes 20 amino acids to grow hair, but our body only produces 11. To obtain the remaining 9 amino acids, you need to have a protein rich diet. If there is protein deficiency in your body, it makes it up by shutting down some processes that require protein to ration it to others. Unfortunately, hair growth is one of those bodily functions that suffers when we don't have enough protein.

But also don't forget fruits and vegetables, as these are the sources of many minerals and vitamins that your body needs to grow hair quickly.

Vitamins are really necessary:

- Vitamin A stimulates the production of sebum. Sebum ensures proper hydration of your hair follicles and skin. This in turn ensures that your hair keeps looking healthy. Great sources of vitamin A include broccoli, eggs, carrots, meat, cheese, liver, pumpkin, and dark green leafy vegetables.

- Vitamin B3, found in food items like wheat, chicken, beef, and fish helps boost circulation, which as we discussed is necessary to carry essential nutrients to your beard. Note that B3 is even more effective when taken with biotin, to which we will return in a while.

- Pantothenic Acid/Vitamin B5 helps the body to efficiently utilize fats and protein. It also helps to reduce stress. Foods to try in this regard include bread (whole-grain), brewer's yeast, broccoli, avocado, egg yolks, mill, lobster, and organ meats etc.

- Vitamin C is one of the most essential components of a strong immune system, which is necessary for healthy hair and skin. Citrus is the most common item associated with vitamin C. Other foods include green peppers, dark green vegetables, potatoes, and tomatoes.

- Vitamin E is yet another nutrient that promotes healthy skin, and it also ensures proper blood flow. Foods rich in vitamin E include oils, leafy vegetables, nuts, and beans. You can also use topical applications that have vitamin E.

- Folic acid not helps your hair to grow thicker, but also aid in its repair. Foods like whole-grain breads and cereals, leafy green vegetables, peas, and nuts are great sources of folic acids.

Biotin and Beard Growth

Not only does biotin metabolizes amino acids and carbohydrates, but this water-soluble B vitamin is necessary for the formation of glucose and fatty acids. If you have biotin deficiency in your body, it will affect hair growth as well. Make sure you get as low as 30 mcg. And while there are many popular biotin supplements, but you should go for food source of this vitamin, such as yeast, cereals, egg yolks, soy flour, carrots, fish, beans, oysters, liver, and cauliflower.

Cutting Back on the Sugars

Growing your beard is fun, but there are some things that you actually need to avoid in order to get that manly stubble. Top of the list is sugar, which actually makes you hair weaker, and hence, eating and drinking items high in sugar make it harder to grow a beard. Of course, there is some sugar content in fruits and dairy products, which you need to consume, but these are less harmful than candy, baked goods, and carbonated beverages.

Stop Smoking

Smoking damages the body's immune system significantly. Thus, when your immune system isn't at its 100%, you will not be able to grow hair as effectively as you desire.

So if you are a chain smoker, you need to cut back on your habit because nicotine reduces the body's ability to absorb essential nutrients like the ones listed above. These nutrients do not reach the hair follicles, and thus their growth is stunted. Not to mention, nicotine also constricts blood vessels, and you already know the dangers of poor blood flow.

Drink Water, Lots of It

Water is life, so drink plenty of it. You need to stay hydrated at all times so that your body is performing optimally, which is necessary for beard growth. Ideally, drink roughly eight 8-oz (250-ml) glasses each day.

Maintaining your Beard

Now that you have started growing your beard and have hopefully managed to create noticeable patch, you can maintain it with style.

The beard grows in stages, and you are free to use variety of styles to enhance its appearances, even if what you have now is just stubble.

Also, if you trim your beard after every 6-7 weeks, you will be able to maintain the appearance of a thicker and full beard. Of course, no one is stopping you from keeping a raw, curly beard, but a little styling does look good, especially if you have to manage formal engagements.

Like all good things in life, good beard maintenance requires spending money. Finding a good stylist or facial groomer is an investment, as he will not only introduce new styles, but also help you grow your beard in the best possible way.

Also remember that some men do find it easy to grow a beard, but the hair comes in distinct patches, leaving some 'blanks' on the face. But fear not, for there are some products out there can help you cover the empty spaces and your beard look fuller and thicker. Your stylist will have such products on hand. Examples include beard thickeners, which are sprays that give you a great look when you use them on thin, patchy growth areas.

Just remember not to overdo this, and also chose a color that resembles your hair color most.

With these aspects covered, here are the essentials of beard maintenance:

Selecting the Right Length

The length of your beard will depend on the style you want to adopt. This in turn allows you select the right trimmer, and other components of your beard maintenance kit (discussed in the next chapter).

There is virtually no upper limit on the length of your beard. You can grow one for the rest of your years, and it will bloom to its maximum length. Of course, at the start, you will keep the beard growing for weeks at length without trimming it significantly. Only after you think that you have reached the desired thickness can you start selecting styles.

Some of the primary considerations for the perfect style include the shape of your jaw, and the face in general. For instance, if your face is thin and you let your beard grow thick, it will make the face appear slightly fat. On the other extreme, maintaining stubble on a thin face will make you look like

Adrian Brody from the *Pianist* which may win you awards, but it will hardly make a dent on your love life.

The key to a great beard look is experimenting constantly. This is yet another benefit of keeping a beard. No matter how much you trim and chip it off, it will keep coming back, and you have a fresh start to try a new look. And once you do find what works best for you, then you need to have a system to sustain it which may involve having a personal maintenance kit and/or visiting a barber more than you visit your dentist.

But in any case, it is better to start slow with your trimmer, keeping it at a high number setting. Running this over your beard will clear off the stray hair while the volume doesn't get affected and simultaneously you avoid cutting the beard too short. Decrease the length slowly until you reach the desired look. Just remember, while the beard grows back, it does so in a couple of days (or weeks). So only if you can make the wait, it is better to reduce it gradually to avoid any accident that leaves your beard too short.

Cheek Line

Just like maintaining the length of the beard, you need to start slow when shaving the beard off your cheeks to see how much hair suits this part of your face. Maintaining the cheek line is not as difficult as the neck line, unless of course you have hair growth all over your face. Other than that, all you really have to do is removing odd hair from your cheeks.

Most men with regular beards maintain their cheek line moderately high to ensure the best look and shape. We advise that you do the same.

Neck Line

The neck line gives your beard that look of completeness. When you cut it too high, you may possibly be looked down upon your brothers in hair. On the other hand, leaving the neck beard free flowing risks it mingling with your chest hair, which is also not a pleasant sight.

The trick is to start low and cut it bit by bit until you see the consistency. This is necessary, for if you cut one side too high, you will have to shave the other side in similar fashion to get even. But then both sides are high, and it now looks like you have a double chin. You can completely shave off the beard to remove this look, or wait patiently for the necessary hair to grow back.

The key is to remember that it is the 'neck' line, and hence, your focus should be one keeping it as far away from the chin and jaw as possible.

Start in the middle with a straight downward shave. From here you work sideways, reaching both ears. Go slowly to maintain symmetry. This of course takes some practice to get it done. Most people prefer to have it done by a professional.

THE BEARD KIT

We have talked a lot of beard maintenance. While you may have dedicated barber or stylist to help you in this respect, a bearded man should never be without his tools. This is especially true when you are travelling, or when those manly whiskers need emergency tweaking. Here are a few tips on assembling a basic beard maintenance kit:

Beard Oil and Conditioners

We have already discussed the benefits of conditioners and oils for your beard. Depending on the season and the growth of your beard, the hairs can harden and even dry out. Plus, when you wash your face with soap or shampoo on a regular basis, the skin can get really dry. Hence, you should always have a bottle of oil or conditioner in handy to soften the beard hair and keep the skin from getting excessively dry.

Aftershave

As you shave some parts of your face and neck clean, you will also need to keep aftershave in your kit. Quality aftershave only to prevents skin irritation (one downside of having beard), but will also soothe the razor burns.

The aftershave is a common beard product, but it is particularly useful for those that adorn a style that requires extra shaving with a razor. Unless you really know you want, refrain from purchasing the aftershave online. It is better that you go to the store and smell it before purchasing it.

Beard Comb

When you get a comb set, you will most probably get a large comb, pocket comb, and then one for beard trimming (and perhaps a moustache comb as well). These combs come in handy to keep your beard 'in order'. The larger comb helps in untangling the beard as it grows longer. On the other hand, the pocket comb helps with day to day upkeep.

The smaller beard trimming comb perhaps has the greatest use. When you are trimming your beard, it helps to even it out before and during the shortening process, ensuring that you get a consistent length.

If the comb set you purchased has a moustache comb as well, it will help you in morning to make sure that the 'stache' falls in line with the beard.

Nose Hair Trimmer

If there is anything that can ruin the look of otherwise well-kept beard, it is nose hair. Which is why it will do you good to keep one or two nose hair trimmers in your grooming kit so that you can clip out and shorten these unsightly things as you spot them.

Of course, the basic trimming can be done with a small scissor as well, but without a doubt, a nose hair trimmer offers a better experience.

Beard Trimmer

If you want to maintain a particular beard style, then you definitely need a beard trimmer to keep a consistent length so that you always looks good.

If you are one of those men whose facial hair tends to grow quickly, your beard length can make you look different if it grows too long, and then in an effort to return to your 'original' look, there is always a chance of trimming it too short. That is why it is necessary that you trim your beard slightly and consistently from time to time. This is where an electric beard trimmer will help you out.

Not all trimmers are built alike, and you can easily find one that has the right length option for you. It is also possible to get a trimmer that comes built in to one adjustable comb.

While there are a dozen options to choose from, electric beard trimmers can be broadly put in two major categories: corded and cordless.

Both have their pros and cons, and there is much benefit in purchasing a model each. The corded one is good because it helps you achieve a more consistent cut because the power to the motor is constant when it is plugged to an outlet. On the other hand, the cordless trimmer is great for travelling.

The trimmer you choose will also depend on your beard growth goals, personal taste, and of course your price range. But the best part is that you can easily find good trimmers to match these needs. You can get everything from a basic trimmer with an attached comb to ones with multiple attachments.

Razor

Last but not least, we have the razor, which can be electric or disposable. These are necessary for those who regularly style their beards as this involves shaving parts of your face and neck down to the skin.

Pay attention to the last line, because while a beard trimmer can help you get a near-clean shave look (especially if you remove the guide comb and just use the blades), it is not as tight as the feel achieved with a razor.

This is true even if you are using a beard trimmer that is double ended and comes with a foil shaver on one end. Sure, you can use this tool in time of emergency, but for the best results, it is better to work with tools designed specifically for the task.

The choice of razor depends on your beard, the frequency with which you do razor shaving, and most importantly your preferences.

Miscellaneous Shopping Tips

This is was a general overview of what any shaving kit should have. When talking about the aftershave, we advised that it is best to buy in person. However, we cannot downplay the convenience of online shopping as well.

The additional benefit is that you can get ready-made kits with all the essentials. But of course, you can purchase each item individually to create a thoroughly customized kit for your thoroughly unique beard.

Whichever option you take, there are some shopping tips that will come in handy. The most important one is that you should read reviews of each product before purchasing it, especially when it comes to the electric equipment. The benefit of buying online is that you get all the information pertaining to a particular item that you need. So do go through the reviews before adding it to your shopping cart.

In similar vein, the internet also helps you find the best discounts on your beard essentials. Look for these to bring your overall beard maintenance bill to a minimum.

But do remember that the goal is not to go for the cheapest item. While budget is a major issue, you have to ultimately purchase what works best for your beard growth.

MEDICAL HELP FOR BEARD GROWTH

If you have used the techniques listed in this eBook but still haven't managed to grow a beard, you may need medical help. There are some effective techniques in this regard, which we will briefly run over. It's beyond the scope of this eBook to discuss these treatments in detail.

Testosterone Therapy

Testosterone is the hormone that gives us our mainly features like the beard. If you cannot grow facial hair, what you may be experiencing is a lack of testosterone. While a healthy diet, sleep, stress reduction, and exercise can regulate the hormone activity in your body, some people may still need testosterone therapy.

This is usually performed through injections or topical applications. Oral treatments are available, but these are known to have serious side effects, which is why we will advise against them.

Also remember that the hormone therapy should closely be monitored by your doctor because there is always the danger of overdose. Too much testosterone is equally as bad for your beard growth as the lack of it.

But in any case, testosterone therapy is not a way to grow your beard fast. It can take as many as 12 months for the testosterone to kick in.

Finally, you can consult a plastic surgeon for the possibility of hair transplantation. As a quick solution, the surgeon can transplant hair follicles from other parts of the body to your face.

Moreover, this surgery is the treatment is simple and usually performed on an outpatient basis. You may experience minor skin irritation, but that is the only inconvenience.

But even surgery is not the quickest solution possible. You may need to wait up to two full years!

CONCLUSION

That's about it!

Hopefully his eBook will help your grow our beard real fast. Before closing, we would like to reiterate the fact that while growing a beard itself isn't that difficult, finding the best style for it does take some time. Don't settle for the average look. You want your beard to stand out, and in turn, it should make you stand out.

For this reason, never be afraid of experimenting. And now that you know how to assemble a beard kit, you can literally get any look you want depending on the volume of your facial hair.

Most importantly, when you are regularly grooming and maintaining your beard, you need to ensure that it doesn't eat up on your time and become just another chore.

Many men do not pay attention to the time it takes to trim their beards to perfection. Shaving everyday with a razor is time consuming, but ultimately it depends on the style of beard that you have maintained. If it is an intricate style that will look odd with the growth of even a few extra hairs, that will become a relatively difficult to maintain.

What you can do is choose a style that is easy to maintain in your lifestyle, and go for the more exquisite looks on special occasions. And there are a hundred styles to try all your life. The sky is the limit!

19494796R00027

Printed in Great Britain
by Amazon